Allergic Building inner Strength

in a Hypersensitive World

MrParhers Abdoul

Copyright

Contents

Introduction

Welcome to "Allergic: Building Inner Strength in a Hypersensitive World." In a world where sensitivities are prevalent, navigating life with allergies can present unique challenges. Whether you're managing food allergies, environmental sensitivities, or other allergic conditions, this book is designed to provide you with guidance, support, and inspiration.

In this introduction, we'll explore the significance of understanding hypersensitivity and the impact it can have on daily life. We'll also provide an overview of allergies, including common triggers and allergic reactions, setting the stage for the journey ahead.

Living with allergies isn't just about avoiding certain foods or substances—it's about cultivating resilience, finding empowerment, and embracing a life of possibility. Throughout the chapters that follow, you'll discover practical strategies for managing allergies, building inner strength, and thriving despite the challenges you may face.

Whether you're newly diagnosed with allergies or have been living with them for years, this book aims to be a valuable resource and companion on your journey toward a healthier, happier life. So let's embark on this journey together, as we explore how to build inner strength in a hypersensitive world.

Understanding Hypersensitivity

Hypersensitivity, also known as allergy, is the body's exaggerated response to a substance that is typically harmless to most people. This heightened sensitivity can manifest in various ways, ranging from mild discomfort to severe allergic reactions.

In this section, we delve into the mechanisms behind hypersensitivity reactions, exploring the immune system's role in identifying and responding to allergens. Understanding the physiological processes involved can provide insight into why certain individuals are more prone to allergies and how these reactions manifest.

Furthermore, we examine the different types of hypersensitivity reactions, including immediate hypersensitivity (Type I), delayed hypersensitivity (Type IV), and other less common forms. By understanding the distinctions between these reactions, readers can gain a deeper appreciation for the complexity of allergic responses.

Ultimately, by enhancing our understanding of hypersensitivity, we can better equip ourselves to manage allergies effectively and minimize their impact on our daily lives.

Overview of Allergies

Allergies are a widespread and growing concern affecting millions of individuals worldwide. In this section, we provide a comprehensive overview of allergies, covering key aspects such as prevalence, types of allergies, common triggers, and associated symptoms.

We begin by discussing the prevalence of allergies, highlighting the increasing rates of allergic conditions in recent years and the significant impact they have on public health. Understanding the scope of the allergy epidemic is crucial for appreciating the importance of effective management and prevention strategies.

Next, we explore the different types of allergies, including food allergies, environmental allergies (such as pollen, dust mites, and pet dander), insect sting allergies, and drug allergies. By recognizing the various categories of allergies, readers can better identify their own triggers and tailor their management approach accordingly.

We then delve into common allergens and their sources, providing insights into the substances and environmental factors that commonly provoke allergic reactions. From peanuts and shellfish to pollen and mold, understanding these triggers is essential for minimizing exposure and reducing the risk of allergic reactions.

Finally, we outline the typical symptoms associated with allergies, which can range from mild to severe and may affect different systems of the body. By familiarizing ourselves with these symptoms, we can better recognize when an allergic reaction is occurring and take appropriate action to address it promptly.

By providing an overview of allergies in this section, we aim to lay the foundation for a deeper understanding of allergic conditions and empower readers to take proactive steps in managing their own allergies effectively.

Chapter 1: Recognizing Allergic Triggers

Identifying Common Allergens

Identifying common allergens is crucial for individuals with allergies to avoid triggers and manage their condition effectively. In this section, we explore some of the most prevalent allergens and their sources, providing readers with valuable insights into potential allergenic substances in their environment.

1. Pollen: Pollen from trees, grasses, and weeds is a common allergen, particularly during the spring and fall seasons. Exposure to pollen can trigger allergic rhinitis (hay fever) and exacerbate asthma symptoms.

2. Dust Mites: Dust mites are microscopic organisms that thrive in household dust. Their feces and body fragments can trigger allergic reactions in sensitive individuals, leading to symptoms such as sneezing, itching, and congestion.

3. Mold: Mold spores are a common allergen found both indoors and outdoors. Mold thrives in damp, humid environments and can trigger allergic reactions in susceptible individuals, especially those with asthma.

4. Pet Dander: Pet dander, which consists of tiny particles of skin shed by pets such as cats and dogs, is a common allergen. Allergic reactions to pet dander can range from mild to severe, depending on the individual's sensitivity.

5. Food Allergens: Common food allergens include peanuts, tree nuts, shellfish, fish, milk, eggs, wheat, and soy. Food allergies can cause a range of symptoms, from mild itching and swelling to life-threatening anaphylaxis.

6. Insect Venom: Stings from insects such as bees, wasps, and fire ants can trigger allergic reactions in some individuals. Severe allergic reactions to insect venom can be life-threatening and require immediate medical attention.

7. Latex: Latex allergy is a reaction to proteins found in natural rubber latex. It can cause symptoms ranging from skin irritation to more severe reactions, such as anaphylaxis.

By identifying these common allergens and understanding where they may be found, individuals with allergies can take proactive measures to minimize their exposure and reduce the risk of allergic reactions.

Understanding Allergic Reactions

Allergic reactions occur when the immune system overreacts to a normally harmless substance, perceiving it as a threat. These reactions can range from mild to severe and can affect different parts of the body. In this section, we explore the mechanisms behind allergic reactions and the different ways they can manifest.

1. Immune Response: When a person with allergies is exposed to an allergen, their immune system produces antibodies called immunoglobulin E (IgE). These antibodies trigger the release of chemicals such as histamine, which cause allergic symptoms.

2. Types of Allergic Reactions: Allergic reactions can be classified into four types based on the immune mechanisms involved. Type I reactions are immediate hypersensitivity reactions, while Type II, III, and IV reactions are delayed hypersensitivity reactions that occur over time.

3. Symptoms: Allergic reactions can affect the skin, respiratory system, gastrointestinal tract, and cardiovascular system. Symptoms may include itching, hives, swelling, sneezing, coughing, wheezing, nausea, vomiting, diarrhea, and in severe cases, anaphylaxis.

4. Anaphylaxis: Anaphylaxis is a severe, life-threatening allergic reaction that requires immediate medical attention. It can cause a sudden drop in blood pressure, difficulty breathing, and loss of consciousness. Anaphylaxis can be triggered by food, insect stings, medications, or latex.

5. Management: Managing allergic reactions involves avoiding known allergens, taking medications such as antihistamines and corticosteroids to relieve symptoms, and carrying an epinephrine auto-injector (such as an EpiPen) for emergency treatment of anaphylaxis.

By understanding the mechanisms and symptoms of allergic reactions, individuals with allergies can better recognize and manage their condition, reducing the risk of severe reactions and improving their quality of life.

Creating Allergy-Safe Environments

Creating allergy-safe environments is essential for individuals with allergies to minimize their exposure to allergens and prevent allergic reactions. In this section, we provide practical tips and strategies for creating safe spaces at home, work, and school.

1. Home Environment:

   - Keep the home clean and free of dust, mold, and pet dander by regularly vacuuming, dusting, and using air purifiers.

   - Use allergen-proof mattress and pillow covers to prevent exposure to dust mites.

   - Wash bedding and curtains in hot water regularly to kill dust mites and remove allergens.

   - Avoid smoking indoors, as smoke can worsen allergic symptoms.

2. Work Environment:

- Inform your employer and coworkers about your allergies and any specific triggers you have.

- Request accommodations such as a clean workspace, air purifiers, and a fragrance-free environment if necessary.

- Keep allergy medications and emergency supplies, such as an epinephrine auto-injector, readily available at work.

3. School Environment:

- Inform school staff, including teachers and nurses, about your child's allergies and provide them with an allergy action plan.

- Work with the school to ensure that allergens are not present in your child's classroom or cafeteria.

- Educate your child about their allergies and how to avoid triggers.

4. Eating Out:

- Inform restaurant staff about your allergies and ask about ingredients in dishes to avoid allergens.

- Choose restaurants with allergy-friendly menus or that are willing to accommodate your dietary needs.

5. Traveling:

   - Research allergy-friendly accommodations and restaurants at your destination.

   - Pack allergy medications, including antihistamines and epinephrine auto-injectors, in your travel kit.

By implementing these strategies and creating allergy-safe environments, individuals with allergies can reduce the risk of allergic reactions and enjoy a safer and more comfortable living, working, and learning environment.

Tips for Managing Allergic Symptoms

Managing allergic symptoms is essential for individuals with allergies to maintain their health and quality of life. In this section, we provide practical tips and strategies for managing common allergic symptoms effectively.

1. Avoid Allergens: The most effective way to manage allergic symptoms is to avoid exposure to allergens. Identify your triggers and take steps to minimize exposure, such as using allergen-proof bedding, keeping windows closed during high pollen seasons, and avoiding pets if you are allergic to them.

2. Use Medications: Over-the-counter and prescription medications can help relieve allergic symptoms. Antihistamines can reduce itching, sneezing, and runny nose, while decongestants can help relieve nasal congestion. Corticosteroids can reduce inflammation and swelling.

3. Use Nasal Irrigation: Nasal irrigation with a saline solution can help clear nasal passages and reduce congestion. This can be especially helpful for individuals with allergic rhinitis.

4. Keep Indoor Air Clean: Use air purifiers with HEPA filters to remove allergens from the air. Keep humidity levels low to prevent mold growth, and use exhaust fans in bathrooms and kitchens to reduce moisture.

5. Wear Protective Gear: When outdoors, wear a mask to reduce exposure to pollen, dust, and other allergens. Wear gloves and long sleeves when gardening to avoid contact with allergenic plants.

6. Monitor Pollen Counts: Stay informed about pollen counts in your area and try to stay indoors when pollen levels are high. Keep windows closed and use air conditioning to filter the air.

7. Create an Allergy Action Plan: Work with your healthcare provider to create an allergy action plan that outlines steps to take in case of an allergic reaction. Make sure family members, friends, and coworkers are aware of your plan.

8. Consider Immunotherapy: If your allergies are severe or not well-controlled with other treatments, your healthcare provider may recommend allergen immunotherapy (allergy shots) to desensitize your immune system to allergens over time.

By following these tips and working closely with your healthcare provider, you can effectively manage your allergic symptoms and lead a healthier, more comfortable life.

Chapter 3: Building Inner Resilience

Cultivating Emotional Strength

Living with allergies can be challenging, both physically and emotionally. Cultivating emotional strength is essential for individuals with allergies to cope with the stress and anxiety that can accompany their condition. In this section, we explore strategies for building emotional resilience and maintaining a positive mindset.

1. Education and Awareness: Educate yourself about your allergies, triggers, and treatment options. Understanding your condition can help you feel more in control and confident in managing it.

2. Mindfulness and Stress Management: Practice mindfulness techniques such as deep breathing, meditation, or yoga to reduce stress and anxiety. Managing stress can help prevent allergic reactions and improve overall well-being.

3. Seek Support: Connect with others who have allergies through support groups or online forums. Sharing experiences and tips with others can provide emotional support and reduce feelings of isolation.

4. Focus on Positivity: Stay positive and focus on what you can control. Keep a gratitude journal, practice positive affirmations, or engage in activities that bring you joy and fulfillment.

5. Set Realistic Goals: Break down tasks into smaller, manageable goals to avoid feeling overwhelmed. Celebrate your accomplishments, no matter how small, to boost your confidence and motivation.

6. Seek Professional Help: If you're struggling to cope with the emotional impact of your allergies, consider talking to a mental health professional. Therapy can provide you with tools and strategies to manage stress and improve your emotional well-being.

7. Maintain a Healthy Lifestyle: Eat a balanced diet, exercise regularly, and get enough sleep to support your overall health and emotional well-being. A healthy lifestyle can help reduce the severity of allergic reactions and improve your resilience.

By cultivating emotional strength and resilience, individuals with allergies can better cope with the challenges they face and lead fulfilling, balanced lives.

Developing Coping Strategies

Living with allergies requires developing effective coping strategies to manage the challenges that come with the condition. In this section, we explore various coping strategies that can help individuals with allergies navigate their daily lives with greater ease and resilience.

1. Education and Awareness: Educate yourself about your allergies, including common triggers and symptoms. Understanding your condition can help you make informed decisions and feel more in control.

2. Allergy Action Plan: Work with your healthcare provider to develop an allergy action plan. This plan should outline steps to take in case of an allergic reaction, including when to use medications and when to seek emergency help.

3. Avoidance Strategies: Identify and avoid allergens as much as possible. This may involve making changes to your environment, such as using allergen-proof bedding, installing air purifiers, and avoiding foods that trigger allergic reactions.

4. Medication Management: Take your medications as prescribed and keep them readily available. This may include antihistamines, decongestants, and epinephrine auto-injectors for severe allergic reactions.

5. Emotional Support: Seek support from friends, family, or a therapist to help you cope with the emotional aspects of living with allergies. Talking about your feelings and experiences can be therapeutic and reduce feelings of isolation.

6. Healthy Lifestyle: Maintain a healthy lifestyle by eating a balanced diet, exercising regularly, and getting enough sleep. A healthy lifestyle can help boost your immune system and reduce the severity of allergic reactions.

7. Stress Management: Practice stress-reducing techniques such as mindfulness, meditation, or yoga to help manage stress and anxiety. Stress can worsen allergic reactions, so finding healthy ways to cope is important

8. Stay Informed: Stay up-to-date with the latest information and research on allergies. This can help you better understand your condition and explore new treatment options.

By developing coping strategies tailored to your individual needs, you can effectively manage your allergies and lead a healthier, more fulfilling life.

Chapter 4: Overcoming Challenges

Dealing with Social Situations and Peer Pressure

Social situations and peer pressure can present challenges for individuals with allergies, particularly when it comes to food-related events or activities. In this section, we explore strategies for navigating social situations and handling peer pressure in a positive and assertive manner.

1. Communicate Clearly: When attending social events, communicate your allergies clearly and assertively to hosts and others involved. Explain your dietary restrictions and politely ask about ingredients in dishes to ensure they are safe for you to consume.

2. Plan Ahead: If you know you'll be attending an event where allergens may be present, such as a restaurant or party, plan ahead by eating beforehand or bringing safe snacks or meals with you. This can help you avoid feeling left out or pressured to eat something that may trigger an allergic reaction.

3. Educate Others: Use social situations as an opportunity to educate others about allergies and the importance of allergen awareness. By raising awareness, you can help create a more inclusive and understanding environment for everyone.

4. Set Boundaries: Be assertive in setting boundaries when it comes to your allergies. Politely decline offers of food that you know are unsafe for you, and don't feel pressured to eat or try something that could put your health at risk.

5. Seek Support: If you're feeling overwhelmed or anxious in social situations, seek support from friends, family, or a support group for individuals with allergies. Talking about your feelings and experiences can help you feel more confident and supported.

6. Focus on the Social Aspect: Instead of focusing solely on food-related aspects of social events, focus on the social interactions and connections you can make. Engage in conversations, participate in activities, and enjoy the company of others without feeling pressured to eat certain foods.

7. Be Prepared for Reactions: Despite your best efforts, allergic reactions can still occur. Always carry your epinephrine auto-injector and any necessary medications with you, and know how to recognize and respond to allergic reactions quickly and effectively.

By implementing these strategies, you can navigate social situations with confidence and assertiveness while managing your allergies effectively.

Managing Stress and Anxiety

Living with allergies can be stressful, as it often involves constant vigilance and careful planning to avoid allergens. In this section, we explore strategies for managing stress and anxiety associated with allergies, helping you maintain a positive mindset and improve your overall well-being.

1. Identify Triggers: Recognize situations or thoughts that trigger stress and anxiety related to your allergies. Understanding your triggers can help you develop coping strategies to manage them effectively.

2. Practice Relaxation Techniques: Engage in relaxation techniques such as deep breathing, meditation, yoga, or progressive muscle relaxation to reduce stress and promote a sense of calm.

3. Stay Informed: Stay informed about your allergies, treatment options, and ways to manage them effectively. Knowledge can help alleviate anxiety and empower you to take control of your health.

4. Maintain a Healthy Lifestyle: Eat a balanced diet, exercise regularly, and get enough sleep to support your physical and mental health. A healthy lifestyle can help reduce stress and improve your resilience to allergens.

5. Seek Support: Talk to friends, family, or a mental health professional about your feelings and experiences related to your allergies. Seeking support can help you feel understood and less alone in managing your condition.

6. Set Realistic Goals: Break tasks into smaller, manageable goals to avoid feeling overwhelmed. Celebrate your accomplishments, no matter how small, to boost your confidence and motivation.

7. Practice Mindfulness: Stay present in the moment and focus on what you can control. Mindfulness can help reduce anxiety and improve your ability to cope with stress.

8. Limit Exposure to Stressful Situations: Try to avoid or minimize exposure to situations that cause you stress or anxiety. This may involve setting boundaries with others or making lifestyle changes to prioritize your well-being.

By implementing these strategies, you can effectively manage stress and anxiety related to your allergies, leading to a healthier and more balanced life.

Chapter 5: Thriving with Allergies

Embracing Self-Care Practices

Self-care is essential for individuals with allergies to maintain their physical and mental well-being. In this section, we explore self-care practices that can help you manage your allergies and improve your overall quality of life.

1. Healthy Eating: Follow a balanced diet rich in fruits, vegetables, whole grains, and lean proteins. Avoiding allergens and eating foods that support your immune system can help reduce allergic reactions and improve your overall health.

2. Regular Exercise: Engage in regular physical activity to strengthen your immune system and reduce stress. Choose activities that you enjoy and can easily fit into your daily routine.

3. Adequate Sleep: Get enough sleep to support your immune system and overall health. Establish a regular sleep schedule and create a relaxing bedtime routine to improve the quality of your sleep.

4. Stress Management: Practice stress-reducing techniques such as deep breathing, meditation, yoga, or mindfulness to reduce stress and improve your resilience to allergens.

5. Hydration: Stay hydrated by drinking plenty of water throughout the day. Proper hydration can help maintain mucous membrane health and reduce allergic symptoms.

6. Allergen Avoidance: Take steps to avoid allergens in your environment, such as using allergen-proof bedding, keeping windows closed during high pollen seasons, and avoiding foods that trigger allergic reactions.

7. Relaxation Techniques: Incorporate relaxation techniques into your daily routine, such as deep breathing exercises, progressive muscle relaxation, or guided imagery, to reduce stress and promote a sense of calm.

8. Connect with Others: Stay connected with friends, family, and support groups for individuals with allergies. Sharing experiences and tips with others can provide emotional support and reduce feelings of isolation.

9. Professional Help: If you're struggling to cope with your allergies or the stress associated with them, consider seeking help from a mental health professional. Therapy can provide you with tools and strategies to improve your coping skills and emotional well-being.

By embracing self-care practices, you can effectively manage your allergies and improve your overall quality of life. Prioritize your health and well-being, and remember to be kind to yourself as you navigate the challenges of living with allergies.

Finding Joy and Fulfillment Despite Allergies

Living with allergies can present challenges, but it's still possible to find joy and fulfillment in life. In this section, we explore ways to focus on the positive aspects of life and find happiness despite the obstacles posed by allergies.

1. Focus on What You Can Control: While you may not be able to control your allergies, you can control how you respond to them. Focus on managing your allergies effectively and finding solutions that work for you.

2. Pursue Your Passions: Don't let allergies hold you back from pursuing activities and hobbies that bring you joy. Look for allergen-free alternatives or find ways to modify activities to accommodate your allergies.

3. Practice Gratitude: Cultivate a sense of gratitude for the things in your life that bring you joy and fulfillment. Keep a gratitude journal or take time each day to reflect on the positive aspects of your life.

4. Stay Connected: Maintain strong relationships with friends, family, and loved ones. Social support can help reduce stress and improve your overall well-being.

5. Engage in Mindfulness: Practice mindfulness techniques such as meditation or yoga to stay present in the moment and reduce stress and anxiety related to your allergies.

6. Volunteer or Give Back: Helping others can be incredibly fulfilling. Look for ways to volunteer or give back to your community, even in small ways.

7. Seek Professional Help: If you're struggling to find joy and fulfillment despite your allergies, consider talking to a mental health professional. Therapy can provide you with strategies to improve your outlook and find happiness in your life.

8. Celebrate Your Successes: Acknowledge and celebrate your achievements, no matter how small. Recognizing your successes can boost your self-esteem and motivation.

By focusing on the positive aspects of your life and finding ways to manage your allergies effectively, you can find joy and fulfillment despite the challenges you may face. Remember that you are not defined by your allergies, and there is still much joy and happiness to be found in life.

Chapter 6: Support Systems and Resources

Seeking Help from Healthcare Professionals

Managing allergies effectively often requires the expertise of healthcare professionals. In this section, we explore the role of healthcare professionals in diagnosing, treating, and managing allergies, and how they can support you in improving your quality of life.

1. Allergists/Immunologists: Allergists and immunologists are specialists trained to diagnose and treat allergic conditions. They can perform tests to identify your specific allergens and develop a treatment plan tailored to your needs.

2. Primary Care Physicians: Your primary care physician can help manage your allergies by providing routine care, prescribing medications, and referring you to specialists when necessary. They can also help coordinate your care with other healthcare providers.

3. Nurses: Nurses play a vital role in allergy care by providing education, administering medications, and assisting with allergy testing and treatment. They can also provide support and guidance on managing your allergies day-to-day.

4. Pharmacists: Pharmacists can provide valuable information about medications used to treat allergies, including how to take them safely and any potential side effects. They can also help you find over-the-counter remedies for allergy symptoms.

5. Mental Health Professionals: Living with allergies can be stressful, and mental health professionals such as psychologists or counselors can help you cope with the emotional impact of your condition. They can provide support, counseling, and strategies for managing stress and anxiety.

6. Dietitians: If you have food allergies, a dietitian can help you develop a safe and nutritious diet that avoids your allergens. They can also provide guidance on reading food labels and identifying hidden allergens in foods.

7. Emergency Medical Personnel: In cases of severe allergic reactions (anaphylaxis), emergency medical personnel such as paramedics and emergency room doctors play a crucial role in providing immediate care and treatment.

8. Support Groups: While not healthcare professionals, support groups for individuals with allergies can provide valuable emotional support, practical tips, and a sense of community.

By seeking help from healthcare professionals, you can receive the support and guidance you need to manage your allergies effectively and improve your quality of life. Working together with your healthcare team, you can develop a comprehensive treatment plan that addresses your specific needs and helps you live well with allergies.

Connecting with Support Groups and Communities

Living with allergies can be challenging, but connecting with support groups and communities can provide valuable support, information, and a sense of belonging. In this section, we explore the benefits of joining a support group and how to connect with others facing similar challenges.

1. Emotional Support: Support groups can provide a safe space to share your experiences, fears, and frustrations with others who understand what you're going through. This can help reduce feelings of isolation and provide a sense of community.

2. Practical Tips and Information: Support groups can offer practical tips and information on managing allergies, such as allergen avoidance strategies, medication management, and coping techniques.

3. Empowerment and Advocacy: Connecting with others in a support group can empower you to advocate for yourself and others with allergies. You can learn about your rights, raise awareness about allergies, and work towards creating a more allergen-aware society.

4. Access to Resources: Support groups often have access to resources such as educational materials, guest speakers, and online forums where you can ask questions and seek advice from others.

5. Building Relationships: Joining a support group can help you build meaningful relationships with others who share your experiences. These relationships can provide ongoing support and friendship.

6. Finding Support Groups: You can find support groups for allergies through local hospitals, clinics, or community centers. Online resources such as social media groups, forums, and websites dedicated to allergies can also be valuable sources of support.

7. Participating in Events and Activities: Many support groups organize events, meetings, or activities where members can connect in person. Participating in these events can help you build relationships and expand your support network.

8. Starting Your Own Group: If you can't find a support group in your area, consider starting your own. You can reach out to local healthcare providers, community centers, or online platforms to connect with others who may be interested in joining.

By connecting with support groups and communities, you can find the support, information, and understanding you need to manage your allergies effectively and improve your quality of life.

Conclusion

Reflecting on Your Allergic Journey

Reflecting on your allergic journey can be a valuable exercise that allows you to gain insights, learn from your experiences, and acknowledge your progress. In this section, we provide prompts to help you reflect on your journey with allergies:

1. When Were You First Diagnosed with Allergies?

- Reflect on your initial reactions and feelings upon receiving your diagnosis.

- How did you cope with the news, and what steps did you take to learn more about your allergies?

2. What Challenges Have You Faced?

- Think about the challenges you've encountered while managing your allergies.

- How have these challenges impacted your life, and what strategies have you used to overcome them?

3. What Have You Learned About Your Allergies?

- Reflect on the knowledge you've gained about your specific allergens and triggers.

- How has this knowledge helped you better manage your allergies and avoid potential reactions?

4. How Have Your Allergies Affected Your Mental Health?

- Consider the emotional impact of living with allergies.

- Have your allergies caused stress, anxiety, or other mental health challenges? How have you coped with these feelings?

5. What Support Have You Received?

- Think about the support you've received from healthcare professionals, family, friends, and support groups.

- How has this support helped you navigate your allergic journey?

6. What Positive Changes Have You Made?

- Reflect on any positive changes you've made in your life as a result of managing your allergies.

- Have your allergies led you to adopt healthier habits or make other positive lifestyle changes?

7. What Are Your Goals Moving Forward?

- Consider your future goals and aspirations in managing your allergies.

- How do you envision your life with allergies in the coming years, and what steps are you taking to achieve your goals?

8. **What Advice Would You Give to Others with Allergies?

- Based on your experiences, what advice would you give to others living with allergies?

- How can others learn from your journey and better manage their own allergies?

Reflecting on your allergic journey can help you gain a deeper understanding of your experiences, identify areas for growth, and appreciate the progress you've made. It can also serve as a source of inspiration and motivation as you continue to navigate life with allergies.

Looking Ahead: Empowered Living with Allergies

As you look ahead to the future, it's important to approach living with allergies with a sense of empowerment and optimism. In this section, we explore ways to embrace empowered living with allergies and take control of your health and well-being:

1. Education and Awareness: Continue to educate yourself about allergies, including new research, treatment options, and ways to manage your condition effectively. Knowledge is empowering and can help you make informed decisions about your health.

2. Advocacy: Advocate for yourself and others with allergies by raising awareness, promoting allergen safety, and advocating for policies that support individuals with allergies. Your voice can make a difference in creating a more allergen-aware society.

3. Self-Care: Prioritize self-care by eating a balanced diet, exercising regularly, getting enough sleep, and managing stress. Taking care of your physical and mental health can help you better manage your allergies and improve your overall well-being.

4. Support Networks: Stay connected with support groups, online communities, and others who understand your experiences. Building a strong support network can provide you with emotional support and valuable resources.

5. Healthy Lifestyle Choices: Make healthy lifestyle choices that support your immune system and overall health. This includes avoiding smoking, limiting alcohol consumption, and maintaining a healthy weight.

6. Allergen Avoidance: Continue to identify and avoid allergens in your environment, and take steps to minimize your exposure to them. This may include using allergen-proof bedding, keeping windows closed during high pollen seasons, and avoiding foods that trigger allergic reactions.

7. Regular Check-ups: Schedule regular check-ups with your healthcare provider to monitor your allergies and ensure your treatment plan is effective. Regular monitoring can help prevent complications and ensure you're receiving the best possible care.

8. Embracing Life: Despite the challenges of living with allergies, embrace life to the fullest. Pursue your passions, engage in activities you enjoy, and focus on the positive aspects of your life.

By embracing empowered living with allergies, you can take control of your health and well-being, advocate for yourself and others, and live a fulfilling and empowered life despite the challenges posed by allergies.

Appendix: Allergy-Friendly Recipes and Tips

In this section, we provide a selection of allergy-friendly recipes and tips to help you enjoy delicious and safe meals while managing your allergies. These recipes are free from common allergens such as peanuts, tree nuts, dairy, eggs, wheat, soy, and shellfish. Always check ingredient labels and consult with your healthcare provider if you have any questions or concerns about specific ingredients.

1. Allergy-Friendly Banana Pancakes:

- Ingredients: 1 ripe banana, 1/2 cup oat flour, 1/2 teaspoon baking powder, 1/4 teaspoon cinnamon, 1/4 cup dairy-free milk.

- Instructions: Mash the banana in a bowl, then add the oat flour, baking powder, cinnamon, and dairy-free milk. Mix until well combined. Heat a non-stick pan over medium heat and pour batter to form pancakes. Cook until bubbles form on the surface, then flip and cook for another minute. Serve with maple syrup or fruit compote.

2. Allergy-Friendly Veggie Stir-Fry:

- Ingredients: 1 cup mixed vegetables (such as bell peppers, broccoli, and carrots), 1 tablespoon olive oil, 2 tablespoons soy sauce (or tamari for gluten-free), 1 teaspoon sesame oil, 1/2 teaspoon ginger, 1/2 teaspoon garlic powder.

- Instructions: Heat olive oil in a large pan over medium heat. Add vegetables and cook until tender. In a small bowl, mix soy sauce, sesame oil, ginger, and garlic powder. Pour over vegetables and stir to coat. Cook for another 2-3 minutes. Serve over rice or quinoa.

3. Allergy-Friendly Banana Ice Cream:

- Ingredients: 2 ripe bananas, sliced and frozen, 1/4 cup dairy-free milk, 1 teaspoon vanilla extract.

- Instructions: Place frozen banana slices, dairy-free milk, and vanilla extract in a blender or food processor. Blend until smooth and creamy. Serve immediately as soft-serve ice cream or freeze for a firmer texture.

4. Allergy-Friendly Trail Mix:

- Ingredients: 1/2 cup dried fruit (such as raisins or cranberries), 1/2 cup sunflower seeds, 1/2 cup pumpkin seeds, 1/2 cup dairy-free chocolate chips.

- Instructions: Mix all ingredients in a bowl. Store in an airtight container for a convenient and allergy-friendly snack.

5. Allergy-Friendly Baked Sweet Potato Fries:

  - Ingredients: 2 large sweet potatoes, peeled and cut into fries, 2 tablespoons olive oil, 1/2 teaspoon paprika, 1/2 teaspoon garlic powder, 1/2 teaspoon salt.

  - Instructions: Preheat oven to 425°F (220°C). In a large bowl, toss sweet potato fries with olive oil, paprika, garlic powder, and salt. Spread fries in a single layer on a baking sheet lined with parchment paper. Bake for 25-30 minutes, flipping halfway through, until fries are crispy and golden brown.

These allergy-friendly recipes are just a starting point. Feel free to modify them to suit your taste preferences and dietary needs. Experiment with different ingredients and flavors to create delicious meals that are safe and enjoyable for you.

References

- American Academy of Allergy, Asthma & Immunology. (n.d.). Tips to Remember: Food Allergy. https://www.aaaai.org/conditions-and-treatments/library/allergy-library/tips-to-remember-food-allergy

- Asthma and Allergy Foundation of America. (n.d.). Food Allergy. https://www.aafa.org/food-allergies/

- Mayo Clinic. (2021, May 13). Allergies. https://www.mayoclinic.org/diseases-conditions/allergies/symptoms-causes/syc-20351497

- National Institute of Allergy and Infectious Diseases. (2017, January). Guidelines for the Diagnosis and Management of Food Allergy in the United States: Report of the NIAID-Sponsored Expert Panel. https://www.niaid.nih.gov/sites/default/files/FoodAllergyGuidelines.pdf

- World Allergy Organization. (n.d.). About Allergy. https://www.worldallergy.org/education-and-programs/education/allergic-disease-resource-center/about-allergy.